The Simple Pregnancy Guide

A Healthy

Manual For First Time Moms

Planning A Stress-Free Delivery

By

Dr. Jane Smart

www.MillenniumPublishingLimited.com

Disclaimer

This publication is designed to provide competent and reliable information regarding the subject matter covered. However, it is sold with the understanding that the author is not engaged in rendering medical or other professional advice. Laws and practices often vary from state to state and country to country and if medical or other expert assistance is required, the services of a professional should be sought. The author specifically disclaims any liability that is incurred from the use or application of the contents of this book.

Books By Dr. Jane Smart

<u>Strong Woman</u>

<u>20 Ways To Rekindle The Love In Your Marriage</u>

<u>50 Telltale Signs Your Man Is Taking You For Granted</u>

<u>20 Things Men Love In Women</u>

<u>Bonus Offer</u>

The kindle edition will be available to you for FREE when you purchase the paperback version from Amazon.com (The US Store)

Download The Audio Versions Along With The Complementary PDF Document For FREE *from Amazon.com*

Table of Contents

Introduction 8

Chapter 1 11
Ten Early Pregnancy Symptoms.................................... 11

Chapter 2 17
Pregnancy Test And Due Date 17
When is the right time to take a pregnancy test? 17
How can you calculate your baby's due date? 19

Chapter 3 22
Antenatal Screening 22
What can an ultrasound scan determine?.................. 23
What blood tests will you have?................................. 24

Chapter 4 30
Nutrition in Pregnancy 30
Foods you should eat during pregnancy..................... 31
12 foods you should avoid during pregnancy.............. 34

Chapter 5 39
Weight Gain and Exercise During Pregnancy................. 39
Exercise During Pregnancy 41
Exercises To Avoid 42
Other do's and don'ts.. 43
Postnatally 44

Chapter 6 46
Embryo and Foetal Development 46
Week 3.. 46
Weeks 4 to 5 46
Week 6.. 47
Week 8.. 47
Week 10.. 48
Week 12.. 48

Weeks 13 to 16 48

Weeks 17 to 20 49

Weeks 21 to 24 50

Weeks 25 to 28 50

Weeks 29 to 32 51

Weeks 33 to 36 52

Weeks 37 to 40 52

Chapter 7 55

Changes During Pregnancy 55

Respiratory System 55

Cardiovascular System 55

Gastrointestinal System 56

Endocrine System 56

Uterus 57

Urinary System 57

Musculoskeletal System 58

Skin 58

Spider veins...59

Varicose vein..59

Stretch marks...59

Breasts 60

Other changes..60

Chapter 8 63

Pregnancy Trimesters...63

First Trimester 63

Second Trimester...64

Third Trimester 65

Chapter 9 69

High Risk Pregnancy 69

Smoking Complications..70

Alcohol 71

Hyperemesis Gravidarum (HG) 71

Gestational Diabetes 72

Pre-eclampsia 73

Ectopic Pregnancy.. 74

Placenta Previa 75

Placental Abruption 76

Premature Labour... 76

Older mums 78

Teen Pregnancy 79

Bed Rest 79

Sex During Pregnancy 80

Chapter 10 .... **84**

What Do I Need to Take Into Hospital **84**

Home Equipment Considerations............................... 87

Chapter 11 .... **93**

48 Frequently Asked Question (With Answers)........... **93**

Conclusion **127**

Introduction

Congratulations, you're pregnant! In approximately nine-month's-time a baby boy or girl will arrive in your life, and the real responsibility begins. Rest assured, this book is aimed at helping you cope: Look upon it as your pregnancy companion. We cover topics from trimesters of pregnancy (pregnancy stages), prenatal care, to dietary do's and don'ts.

There is a lot to contend with whilst pregnant and it helps to be prepared. This book is aimed at all mums-to-be. No two pregnancies are the same, and some may have issues to overcome e.g. nausea and vomiting, so it can be useful to have helpful information to hand. Pregnancy is an exciting journey and you are probably more prepared than you realise. If not, this book will provide you with facts around 'what to expect when you are expecting'.

The terms pregnant and prenatal are derived from the Latin words pre - meaning before, and (g)natus - meaning birth. Therefore 'before gives birth'. You may also hear health professionals use the term gestation. This is the period or process, from conception to birth, of the baby developing in the womb.

Pregnancy officially starts from the first day of a woman's last normal menstrual period, even though the development of the fetus does not begin until conception, which is two weeks later. This is because every time you have a period your body is preparing for pregnancy. It also serves as a gauge for health professionals, as it is difficult for them to know precisely when conception occurred. Your expected delivery date is therefore calculated 40 weeks and from the first day of your last period.

Pregnancy consists of three trimesters: First, second and third, which are roughly three months in duration. For the first 10 weeks of your pregnancy (or 8 weeks after conception) your baby is referred to as an embryo. From 10-weeks onwards your baby is known as a foetus. A baby is considered full term from the beginning of the 39th to the end of the 40th week of pregnancy. Typically, a woman will give birth between her 39th and 42nd week, when the pregnancy is left to progress naturally.

Please note: this book is in no way a replacement for the professional care a midwife or doctor can provide. So please talk to them if anything is concerning you

Moses Basket & Bedding Set

Woven from pure Moroccan palm leaf, the Moses Basket has been a popular baby bedding solution for centuries and offers baby a comfortable and secure alternative to bassinets and cradles. Recommended for use with newborns up to 15 lbs or 3 months, the Moses basket keeps baby close at hand during an afternoon or evening snooze.

Once your baby outgrows the basket, turn the baby basket into a laundry or storage basket! Warning: Moses basket is NOT for carrying baby; make sure baby is out of the basket before it is picked up or moved.

To Learn More, Go to

www.MillenniumPublishingLtd > Dr-Jane-Smart >
Pregnancy Required Items

Chapter 1

Ten Early Pregnancy Symptoms

There are a variety of symptoms you may experience during early pregnancy. Not all women experience the same ones, and they can differ with successive pregnancies. Some can appear when you have missed a period, others not for a few weeks. Here are a few:

1. A missed period

Women that have regular periods, but then miss one may do a pregnancy test before any other symptoms occur. For others with irregular periods, the first inkling they might be pregnant could be breast tenderness, nausea or needing the loo more often!

2. Fatigue

You might not just feel sleepy, you may be exhausted! Although no one is sure, it may be the increase of the hormone progesterone that makes you feel tired. Obviously, if you need to wee more often and you feel sick, this can add to the tiredness. Women usually start to have more energy once into the 2nd trimester. Tiredness will usually return in late pregnancy, when the weight of the baby can make it harder for you to get a good night's sleep. Be sure to rest when the chance arises and accept help if it is offered. Remember housework can wait, looking after yourself comes first!

3. Abdominal bloating

As with a period, the hormones associated with early pregnancy can make you feel bloated. So even though there is no outward sign of pregnancy your clothes may feel a little tight.

4. A frequent need to urinate

Hormonal changes in pregnancy mean that the blood flow to your kidneys increases. This means your bladder fills more quickly, which in turn makes you urinate more often! This frequent need to wee increases later in pregnancy, when the baby's weight puts more pressure on your bladder.

5. Food aversion

It can be common for women in early pregnancy to feel nauseated when confronted with certain smells e.g. coffee, spicy food. It can often be things that you really enjoyed prior to pregnancy. Strong smells may even make you want to gag. Although experts do not know for certain why this occurs, it may be due to the increasing amount of oestrogen in your system.

6. Sore breasts

Rising hormone levels can cause sensitive swollen breasts, again like before a period. This should ease after your first trimester, as your body becomes more used to the hormonal changes

7. Mood swings

These are common in early pregnancy, and are due to hormone changes that effect the chemical messengers in your brain. Some mums-to-be may feel a positive effect, others may feel depressed or anxious. If you are finding it hard to cope, make sure to contact your healthcare provider immediately.

8. Elevated basal temperature

Your basal temperature is the lowest measurement of your body's temperature, when taken first thing in the morning. Some women chart their temperature, to establish when they are due to ovulate, and therefore more likely to conceive. If it remains high for over 2 weeks, then you are likely pregnant.

9. Spotting

It is natural to feel concerned, if after wanting to be pregnant, you then see bleeding. If this happens around the time you would normally have a period, it could be due to implantation bleeding, i.e. the fertilized egg settling in the lining of your womb. If the bleeding is severe, accompanied by pain, or you just need reassurance, contact your midwife or doctor.

10. Nausea and/or vomiting

Commonly known as 'morning sickness'. It usually starts at about 8 weeks into pregnancy, but for some women it can appear as early as 2 weeks. It can also occur any time of day or night. Nausea will normally begin to ease by the start of the 2nd trimester. Some of the following may mean you are at more risk of developing nausea and vomiting.

- A first pregnancy.
- Multiple pregnancy e.g. twins or triplets.
- Nausea and vomiting in a previous pregnancy.
- A family history of nausea and vomiting in pregnancy. For example, if your mum experienced morning sickness carrying you, you may find you will too!

- If you have experienced nausea when using contraceptives that contain oestrogen.

- If you suffer from motion sickness: for example, travelling in a car.

- Being obese, with a body mass index (BMI) of 30 or more.

- Stress.

We cover what you can do to help nausea and vomiting in the Q & A section at the end of this book.

Baby Changing Table

Changing tables give you a much needed helping hand. With safety belts, rails and shelves, you can keep necessary items within arm's reach so you're never tempted to leave your baby unattended. This particular changing table is also design to be at a comfortable height so that it's easy to swoop in for some baby nuzzling.

To Learn More, Go to

www.MillenniumPublishingLtd > Dr-Jane-Smart >

Pregnancy Required Items

Chapter 2

Pregnancy Test And Due Date

Many home pregnancy tests are not sensitive enough to detect you are pregnant until approximately a week after you've missed a period. If it shows a negative result, wait a few days and try again. Looking after your health is vital, even if you don't have a positive result yet.

When is the right time to take a pregnancy test?

There are different pregnancy tests available, depending on the timing of conception and your preference; There is the classic urine test and a blood test. The hormone present in your body during pregnancy is called human chorionic gonadotrophin (hCG). It is produced by the placenta shortly after the embryo attaches to the wall of the uterus, and can usually be detected in urine six to twelve days after the egg has been fertilized. The hCG produced doubles every two to three days.

It is advisable to wait until the first day of your missed period to take a pregnancy test. This ensures that the level of hCG is high enough to be detected. It is recommended you take a pregnancy test using the first urine of the day, due to the urine being more concentrated, therefore the hCG level is easier to detect.

A blood test can be taken by your midwife or doctor. It also detects the presence of the hormone, hCG and can be performed six to eight days after ovulation. There are two types of blood tests: Qualitative and quantitative. A qualitative test gives a simple yes or no answer to whether you are pregnant or not. The quantitative tests, also known as beta hCG, shows the exact level of hormone found in your blood.

If you think you are pregnant but received a negative result with your home pregnancy test, don't worry. False-negatives can occur due to a variety of factors: The urine was too dilute to detect hCG; the test was done incorrectly or you tested too soon, or home pregnancy test has passed its use by date. Fertility medication, or other drugs containing hCG can interfere with home pregnancy tests. However, other medications, such as antibiotics or birth control pills shouldn't.

It is rare, but false-positives do occur and can be due to blood or protein being present in your urine. Certain drugs, such as anticonvulsants or tranquilisers can also cause false-positive test results.

Whether you have received a positive or negative result with a home pregnancy test, it is always best to seek the advice of a medical professional as soon as possible.

How can you calculate your baby's due date?

Women do not have identical menstrual cycles; and if you have irregular periods your due date may be difficult to pinpoint. However, if you have a regular menstrual cycle of 28 days, you can estimate a due date by adding 280 days (9 months, 7 days) to the first day of your last period. Please remember this is not always 100% accurate and should be taken as an estimate only.

Your last menstrual period and ovulation are included in the first two weeks of your pregnancy. This may seem strange, as it means you are officially pregnant before you conceive! Only 5% of babies are born on their due date. 80% of women deliver somewhere between 37 and 42 weeks, which means approximately 15% deliver prematurely. Although there may not always be an obvious reason, there are certain risk factors that mean you may go into labour early e.g. multiple pregnancy, infection.

If you are a woman that has irregular periods, how can you determine your due date? First, if you can remember the date of your last menstrual cycle you can still use the calculation above. Another way for a midwife to estimate your baby's due date is to palpate your abdomen. They assess the fundal height: this is the top of the uterus (which reaches your navel at around 20 weeks.) An ultrasound scan can also be performed to determine your expected due date, if other methods have not worked or your midwife wants to confirm it.

A caesarean section is an alternate way to give birth and your due date may not be the only thing to consider, if one is required. They are usually scheduled no sooner than 7 days before your due date.

However, and whenever your baby is born, enjoy the moment. Many women would tell you, babies usually come when they are ready, and remember a due date is just an estimate!

Baby Monitor

A Smart Baby monitor gives you a good view of your baby day and night. You can see and hear your baby 24/7 with HD live streaming, unparalleled night vision, and zoom to get in close. This particular monitor also works over Wi-Fi, even when internet is down!

To Learn More, Go to
www.MillenniumPublishingLtd > Dr-Jane-Smart > Pregnancy Required Items

Chapter 3

Antenatal Screening

Screening is an important part of pregnancy. When to test and what tests to have are important questions; and whether you are pregnant with your first child or been pregnant before, any testing can be nerve-wracking. Antenatal screening is carried out in all three trimesters. Each test is important, as they help assess both you and your baby's health, at different stages of your journey.

Hospitals in the UK offer all pregnant women at least two ultrasound scans during pregnancy. There are no known risks to either you or your baby, but it is important to make sure you have all the facts before having an ultrasound. If you choose not to go ahead, your choice will be respected, and you can continue with all other aspects of antenatal screening. Talk to you midwife/doctor about your concerns.

What can an ultrasound scan determine?

- Your baby's size. The dating scan will give you a better idea of how many weeks pregnant you are.
- Whether you are having one, or more babies.
- It can detect some abnormalities.
- The position of the baby and the placenta. If they find that the placenta is low, later in pregnancy, it may mean you are advised to have a caesarian section.
- To make sure that the baby is growing as expected. This is important for all pregnancies, but considered more so if you're carrying twins or you have experienced problems in this or a previous pregnancy.

The first ultrasound is carried out at 8 to 14 weeks, and is used to confirm your due date, based on your baby's measurements. The scan usually lasts about 20 minutes, but don't worry if the sonographer can't get a good view. It is normally because the baby is moving around, or is in an awkward position. Also, the ultrasound quality may not be as clear, if you are overweight or your body tissue is dense. It may take longer for the ultrasound, or you may need to have a repeat scan. The sonographer may also do what is known as a 'nuchal translucency test'. This is part of the screening test for Down Syndrome.

The second ultrasound is carried out at 18 to 21 weeks, and is used to detect abnormalities or irregularities. Some women may have more than two scans, and this is usually due to either an issue with their health, or the health of their baby. Someone can accompany you to the scan, although you may not want to take young children with you. If you want to know the sex of the baby, you can usually do so at the 18 to 21-week scan.

NB: It is not always possible for the sonographer to confirm the baby's sex, and some hospitals may have a policy of not telling you. Ask your midwife or sonographer for more information.

What blood tests will you have?

Blood tests are a routine part of antenatal care, and they give you and your midwife or doctor important information on your health, and that of your baby. At your first booking appointment, you will be offered some, or all these tests. If you don't understand what a certain test is for, ask your midwife or doctor to explain. As with a scan, only you can decide if you want to have the blood tests:

1. Blood Group

This is in case you require a blood transfusion during pregnancy, or labour.

2. Haemoglobin

This detects whether the level of haemoglobin in your blood is low, which means you have iron deficiency anaemia. Your body needs iron to produce haemoglobin, which in turn carries oxygen around your body in red blood cells. If you are anaemic, your midwife/doctor will advise what foods eat to boost your iron levels. They may also prescribe iron tablets.

3. Rhesus Factor

If a person's blood shows that they are rhesus positive, it means they have a certain protein on the surface of their red blood cells. If you are rhesus negative but the baby's father is rhesus positive, there is a chance the baby will be positive too. If this is the case, your body may start to produce antibodies that attack the baby's red blood cells. You can be given an injection of an antibody called immunoglobulin, at 28 weeks. Ask your midwife/doctor for more details

4. Hepatitis B

If you pass hepatitis B on to your baby, before or after they are born, they need to be started on a series of injections (vaccine and antibodies) as soon as they are born. Your doctor will carry out a blood test, when your child reaches one, to see if they have avoided infection.

5. Syphilis

Thankfully this sexually transmitted disease is rare nowadays. But if you do have it and it isn't treated, while you are pregnant, it could cause abnormalities in your baby. Syphilis can also cause a baby to be stillborn. The blood test can sometimes produce a false-positive result. This is because the syphilis bacteria and other bacteria (that cause non-sexually transmitted diseases) can look similar. If you do have syphilis, you will be treated with penicillin. This might be enough to prevent your baby from contracting the disease but some may need antibiotics after birth.

6. HIV/AIDS

All mums-to-be are offered a blood test to detect HIV/AIDS. You can turn it down if you want to. However, if the doctors know you have the virus, steps can be taken to reduce the chance of the virus being transmitted to your baby.

Blood Tests for Other Disorders

In most cases, sickle-cell disorders are more likely in people of African and African-Caribbean descent, while Thalassaemia is more common in people of Asian or Mediterranean origin. If you come from these backgrounds you should be offered a test for sickle-cell or thalassaemia at your booking appointment. They can make you anaemic, and can be passed on to your baby. In most parts of the UK, all pregnant women are offered a test for thalassaemia. But there are different approaches to screening for sickle-cell disease, depending on how prevalent the condition is in the area. All pregnant women should be offered screening, in areas where there is a high number of cases.

Furthermore, all pregnant women should be offered a screening test for genetic abnormalities e.g. Down syndrome. One of the most accurate tests is the combined screening test. This consists of blood tests and the nuchal translucency scan, mentioned earlier, that is done at your dating scan. This is now recommended throughout the UK, as it gives a more reliable risk rating (whether your baby may have problems).

Screening tests can't tell you 100% that your baby has a problem. If you want to be certain, you need to go on to have diagnostic tests such as chorionic villus sampling or amniocentesis. These will be discussed with you if it is found on the combined screening test that your baby may have problems.

Not all women need all blood tests. Many factors come into play when deciding what and when to test. You need to discuss with your midwife/doctor which tests are right for you.

Baby Bouncer

Everyone needs their own happy place. This infant bouncer is made just for your little one: a babies-only hangout where the only ticket to entry is adorableness. Spin up sweet moments with the colorful pinwheel design, and keep baby calm with smooth vibrations. One happy baby! A toy bar hangs above your baby with cheerful toys that spin and spin. When you're ready to scoop up your baby, the toy bar easily removes. With a lightweight and portable design, baby's happy place can be with you.

To Learn More, Go to

www.MillenniumPublishingLtd > Dr-Jane-Smart > Pregnancy Required Items

Chapter 4

Nutrition in Pregnancy

A healthy diet should be a part of daily life, whether pregnant or not. Nutrition plays an important role in pregnancy, and you need to remember the foetus is connected to you by the placenta and receives all its nutrients via the umbilical cord.

If you have any specific dietary concerns based on factors such as religious/ethical beliefs; medical issues (e.g. allergies), please make an appointment to see your health professional prior to, or as soon after conception as possible. They can then help you plan a healthy diet, tailored to your specific needs or refer you to a dietician if necessary.

Above all, you need to follow a healthy diet and your body needs extra vitamins and minerals but there is no need to 'eat for two'. It is advised that you eat an extra 350 to 500 calories (1470 to 2090 kilo-joules) during the 2nd and 3rd trimesters only. If your diet is lacking, it may affect the baby's development, also poor eating habits and excess weight gain puts you at higher risk of gestational diabetes, or birth complications.

It is important that your baby gets a good supply of nutrients.

Foods you should eat during pregnancy

The following 5 foods should make up the basis of your healthy diet.

1. Fruits and vegetables

There are vitamins, minerals and fibre in fruits and vegetables, that ensure healthy growth in your baby, and aid digestion and prevent constipation in you. It is advised you eat at least 5 portions of fruit and vegetables a day. Leafy green vegetables such as broccoli and kale contain folate and vitamin B6. You should have been taking folic acid prior to pregnancy and up until week 12, and you may be taking antenatal vitamins that contain folic acid (folate).

However, eating foods containing folate is a plus. Other fruit and veg that contain folate and vitamin B are: Citrus fruits, dried beans, peas. Make sure you always wash fruit and vegetables carefully. If abroad wash them using bottled or cooled, boiled water, as the tap water may be contaminated.

2. Protein

Needs to be a part of your daily diet. Sources of protein include fish, meat (avoid liver), poultry, eggs, beans, pulses and nuts. Choose lean meat and remove the skin for poultry when cooking, and try to use little or no oil when cooking. You need to make sure that all meat, fish, eggs etc. are cooked thoroughly. If you can, eat at least 2 portions of fish a week (one should be an oily fish like mackerel). Please see the section below for meat to avoid.

3. Carbohydrates (starchy foods)

These are important for energy, certain vitamins and fibre. They should make up a third of your diet and can help fill you up, and if you choose wisely should not contain too many calories. These include bread, potatoes, breakfast cereal, pasta, oats and rice. Swap refined, white options for wholegrain, high fibre options.

4. Dairy Foods

Milk, cheese, yoghurt etc. are important in pregnancy as they provide you and baby with calcium. Try to choose lower fat options (you still receive the required amount of calcium). If you do not eat dairy you can substitute with soya drinks etc. Please see the section below for cheeses to avoid in pregnancy.

5. Iron

Legumes such as, lentils, kidney beans, black beans and chick peas, are a great source of iron. You and your baby use a lot iron during pregnancy, and it is important to keep replenishing the supply. It is better to consume iron in food, than to take iron supplements, as these can lead to constipation.

Some foods (high in fat and sugar) should be consumed in moderation throughout your pregnancy, as they can lead to excess weight gain. This is not good for either you or your baby, as it can lead to pregnancy complications, like gestational diabetes. These include but are not limited to: Oils; spreads (margarine or butter); chocolate; crisps; cake; biscuits; deserts. No-one is saying they should be completely banned but they should be consumed less often and in small amounts!

12 foods you should avoid during pregnancy

It is recommended you do not eat the following:

1. Certain cheese

Soft pasteurised cheeses e.g. camembert, mozzarella. These can contain listeria (a bacteria) that can harm your unborn baby. Stick to eating hard cheese varieties, like cheddar or edam.

2. Cream and custard

You should avoid pre-prepared foods e.g. bakery items with custard or cream used as an ingredient. Also, avoid ready-made supermarket custard.

3. Hummus

It is best to avoid store bought hummus and other pre-packaged, chilled dips. They may contain bacteria that are harmful to your baby. Homemade hummus/dips are generally considered safe. Just ensure you store them in the fridge (in an air-tight container) and use within a couple of days.

4. Pate

This too can contain listeria (vegetable pâté isn't safe either.)

5. Raw or partially cooked eggs

Eggs can contain salmonella, which is a major cause of food poisoning. When pregnant, avoid any food that contains uncooked egg e.g. homemade mayonnaise. You don't need to avoid eggs completely, as they're a great source of protein. Just make sure that both the yolk and white are well cooked.

6. Raw, cured and undercooked meat

Raw, undercooked, or cured meats like ham and pepperoni, increase the risk of food poisoning and parasitic infections, and can affect your baby's development. You also need to be extra careful how you cook chicken, as it can contain salmonella and other bacteria. It should be well cooked, all the way through. Be careful of smoked salmon, as it hasn't been through traditional cooking processes and can carry bacteria. It's a good idea to avoid this during pregnancy.

7. Liver

Liver contains high levels of Vitamin A, which in large quantities can harm your baby. You need to be careful with vitamin or mineral supplements during pregnancy. If you think you need supplements, discuss this with your GP.

8. Some types of fish

Fish is a fantastic source of vitamins, minerals and protein, and is also high in omega 3 fatty acids, which help your baby's nervous system develop. Most common types of fish are safe. However, some contain higher levels of Mercury and other pollutants. If you have any doubts about whether a type of fish is safe to eat please talk to your midwife/doctor or see a dietician.

9. Raw shellfish

Reduce the risk of food poisoning by not eating raw shellfish and making sure any shellfish you do eat is thoroughly cooked.

10. Pre-prepared chilled meals and leftovers

Keep all cooked foods in the fridge and ensure you cook them at high temperatures to kill bacteria. The food should be piping hot right the way through.

11. Caffeine

Drinking an excess of caffeine can lead to low birth weight, and it has also been linked to miscarriages. It is best to limit your intake of caffeine or alternatively choose decaffeinated versions of your favourite hot drinks. Pregnant and breastfeeding women are advised to limit their caffeine intake to a maximum of 300mg per day. This is roughly equivalent to 4 cups of plunger coffee, 6 cups of instant coffee, or 6 cups of tea, or 400g plain chocolate!

12. Sushi

It is best to avoid sushi made with raw fish, while trying to conceive or pregnant. Raw fish can contain bacteria and viruses that are harmful to you and your baby. Stick to sushi made with cooked meat or vegetables.

Pram

This exceptional multipurpose carriage, stroller, and car seat combo is a durable travel stroller that includes the Sarema Infant Car Seat and Safe Zone Base. The Sarema Infant Car Seat features an anti-rebound bar that limits the amount of rebound movement experienced by baby in a frontal impact.

To Learn More, Go to
www.MillenniumPublishingLtd > Dr-Jane-Smart >
Pregnancy Required Items

Chapter 5

Weight Gain and Exercise During Pregnancy

Pregnancy can make the fittest of us conscious of our size, especially if they are having a multiple pregnancy. Not every body type is the same and weight gain differs from woman to woman. Before pregnancy a woman fits into a specific category with regards to their weight. It depends on a woman's pre-pregnancy weight and Body Mass Index (BMI), how much weight should be gained during pregnancy. Below shows a woman's pre-pregnancy BMI, and their estimated weight gain.

Pre-pregnancy BMI	BMI	Total weight gain
Underweight	Less than 18.5	13kg to 18kg (28lb to 40lb)
Normal weight	18.5 to 24.9	11.5kg to 16kg (25lb to 35lb)
Overweight	25 to 29.9	7kg to 11.5kg (15lb to 25lb)
Obese	30 or more	5kg to 9kg (11lb to 20lb)

NB: This is for women who are experiencing a single pregnancy.

You will read different advice, telling you the average weight gained, in each stage of pregnancy. Some women may put on the most weight during the first 20 weeks. while others will only gain a few kilograms up until 16 weeks, then put on most in the middle of their pregnancy. All women are different and a woman's overall weight gain (carrying a single baby) can be as little as 8kg, or as much as 20kg, with an average of 12 to 14kg. Pregnancy weight gains is broken down into these factors:

- Baby: 3 to 4kg
- Uterus: 1kg
- Amniotic fluid: 1kg
- Placenta: 0.5kg
- Increase in blood volume: 1.5kg
- Breasts: 0.5kg
- Fat stored in preparation for breast feeding: 3.5kg
- Fluid retention: 1.5kg

Once your baby is born, breastfeeding can help you lose some of the baby weight, but keep in mind that it can normally take up to a year to lose all the baby weight.

Exercise During Pregnancy

Exercise is an important part of life, and just as an important part of a healthy pregnancy. In moderation and with some exceptions, exercise you did before becoming pregnant can continue to be enjoyed throughout pregnancy. So, if you were not a marathon runner before becoming pregnant, now is probably not the time to start! Always talk to your midwife or doctor about exercising, whilst pregnant. When exercising, it is important to keep hydrated and be sensible. Skipping meals is never a good idea when pregnant. Your baby needs extra nutrients, so it is better to skip a workout than a meal.

There are a variety of exercises, appropriate to participate in whilst pregnant. So, if you enjoy swimming, walking, yoga, and Pilates, you will benefit from continuing these in pregnancy. As your pregnancy progresses your body may tell you to slow down, a hint you may need to stop the Zumba classes!

Not all exercise is advised during pregnancy. Although there may not be direct evidence to advise against a particular form of pregnancy, it is often due to the fact that the particular exercise puts you more at risk or falls or other injury. These can include, but are not limited to, the following:

Exercises To Avoid

1. Bikram yoga (Hot yoga)

This is done in a heated environment. There hasn't been any specific research done to find out its effects. It is advised that you avoid doing exercise that raises your core body temperature more than 2 degrees Centigrade. This will reduce the chance of neural tube defects e.g. spina bifida

2. Horse riding, gymnastics and cycling

As pregnancy progresses your centre of gravity changes due to your baby bump. You are at an increased risk of falling, so you are advised to avoid these forms of exercise, and any other activities that may put you at risk (e.g. climbing ladders).

3. Contact sports

For example, football, martial arts, hockey. These put you at risk because you may receive a direct blow to your bump, which may cause injury to the baby.

4. Scuba diving

This needs to be avoided during pregnancy, as your baby is not protected against getting decompression sickness ('the bends') or a gas embolus (bubble in the blood, that may cut off the blood supply, or cause difficulty breathing). Scuba diving has been linked to birth defects.

Other do's and don'ts

- Don't position your 'baby bump' in any awkward positions.
- You will probably want to avoid lying flat after 16 week. Your 'bump' will press on blood vessels, reducing cardiac (heart) output. You may feel dizzy and the blood flow to the baby is affected. Try laying on your side.
- You should not participate in any activity where you hold your breath.

- Do not exercise in heat or humid conditions

NB: If you experience any bleeding or cramping while exercising stop immediately, and contact your health professional.

Postnatally

The first six weeks after delivery should be reserved for healing. You may be feeling very tired, so don't do too much, too soon. Try to wait until after your postnatal check, at between six and eight weeks after the birth, before taking up any exercise other than walking.

A Caesarian section is a major operation! You should not push yourself too soon. Again, the first six weeks are needed for healing, and you should not do any strenuous exercise in the first couple of months. Even heavy lifting at home should be avoided.

Breastfeeding Pillow

A lot of new moms consult with lactation specialists after becoming exasperated and exhausted, feeling they should instinctively know how to breastfeed their own baby, and not understanding why they're having trouble. This particular breastfeeding pillow is designed to give moms the confidence they need to feel secure and position them for breastfeeding success. It'll help alleviate stress and demystify what many new mothers and fathers experience during those first precious months of your newborn baby's life.

To Learn More, Go to
www.MillenniumPublishingLtd > Dr-Jane-Smart >
Pregnancy Required Items

Chapter 6

Embryo and Foetal Development

You and your baby's development will be ongoing for the next nine months but we can break it down a little. Remember your weeks of pregnancy are dated from the first date of your last period, so for the first week or so you are not actually pregnant.

Week 3

You will release an egg about 2 weeks after your last period. During week 3 the fertilized egg moves along the fallopian tube towards your womb (uterus). It starts off as a single cell but divides over and over. When it reaches your uterus, it is about 100 cells called an embryo, and implants in the womb lining.

Weeks 4 to 5

This is usually when women suspect they may be pregnant. The embryo is now two layers of cells and about 2mm long. In the outer layer is a hollow tube that has a groove/folds that develops into the brain and spinal cord. The nervous system is starting to develop, as are the foundations that will be the baby's heart and circulatory system. They also have some of their own blood vessels, and are connected to you by some that will go on to become the umbilical cord.

Week 6

There is a bulge where the heart is and a bump at one end. This bump becomes the brain and head. Your baby's face will begin to take shape, there are dimples where the ears will be, and a slight thickening in the place where their eyes are.

Week 8

The embryo is now called a 'foetus' (which means offspring in Latin), weighs 1 gram and is 1.6 cm in length and starts to move around inside your uterus. The nerve cells continue to multiply, and the nervous system begins to form. The inner ear starts to develop but it takes another few weeks for the outer ear to do so. The buds where arms and legs will be, grow longer, and start to form cartilage.

Week 10

By now your baby's face is starting to form, as the eyes are bigger and more noticeable. The mouth has developed with a tongue that has tiny taste buds, and ears start to develop at the side of the head. Hands and feet are developing and there are fingers and toes, but these are webbed in appearance. All the major organs continue to develop, and the heart is fully formed and beats about 180 times a minute.

Week 12

Your baby is around 5.4 cm and weighs 14 grams. All their limbs, bones, organs, muscles and sex organs are in place. Their eyelids remain closed and won't open for a few more months. Up until now the bones have been formed of cartilage but now bone begins to develop. From now on, they need to mature and grow.

Weeks 13 to 16

By the end of week 16 your baby will weigh about 140g and be 13cm approximately. The sex organs on the inside are fully developed and the genitals now start to form externally. They start to swallow amniotic fluid, and their kidneys begin to work, so fluid will pass back into the fluid as urine. Their eyes begin to be sensitive to light, and although they remain closed they can register if there is bright light. The nervous system has continued to develop, along with muscle control. They can now reach with their hands and even grasp them together.

Weeks 17 to 20

By the end of 20 weeks they weigh about 300g and are approximately 27cm long. Their facial features take on a more human appearance and they have eyelids and eyebrows. They can move their eyes but their eyelids remain closed. Fingerprints are now present, making them a unique person, and finger and toe nails are growing. Baby is now moving around a lot, and this is when you may start to feel them. A lot of women say it feels like 'butterflies in their tummy', its official term is 'quickening'. They will respond to loud music or bangs. They continue to put on weight throughout but at this stage they don't have much of a fat store, so appear a little wrinkled. 'Vernix' appears at around 20 weeks, which is a waxy like substance, that can help to protect newborns from infection. It contains antioxidants, anti-inflammatory and antibacterial properties.

Weeks 21 to 24

At the end of 24 weeks, your baby will weigh approximately 660 grams and be 34.6cm long. From now onwards they will weigh more than the placenta. They develop a more defined waking and sleep pattern, and unfortunately this is not always the same as you! Their lungs are not yet full formed but they start to practice breathing for when they are born. They are covered in a soft, very fine hair which is called 'lanugo'. It is not 100% known why it is present but may have something to do with temperature regulation, and it usually disappears before birth.

Weeks 25 to 28

Your baby will weigh 1.15kg at the end of 27 weeks, and they continue to put on weight, due to fat now appearing under their skin. Their systems are fully formed but need time to mature. Your midwife/doctor will be able to hear their heartbeat through a stethoscope, and it will beat at about 100 beats each minute. They will now move rapidly and may respond to your touch. Their eyelids open around this time and they start blinking. They continue to swallow the amniotic fluid, produce urine and may start to get hiccoughs (hiccups), which you may feel!

Weeks 29 to 32

By the end of 32 weeks they will be approximately 1.92kg and 44cm in length. Your baby continues to be very active, and you will become aware of their patterns in movement. Every baby has their own pattern, so don't worry if yours differs to another pregnant woman. The vernix and lanugo start to decrease in amount. Their sucking reflex has now started to develop, so they can suck their fingers or thumb, and their eyes can focus. The lungs continue to develop but they are not usually able to breathe unaided until they reach 36 week's gestation. By this time, you may find your baby turns to face downward, in readiness for birth. This is known as a 'cephalic presentation'. Don't be concerned if they haven't, as there is still time.

NB: If you notice any change in your baby's movement pattern or you have any concerns, contact your GP/Midwife.

Weeks 33 to 36

By the end of week 36 your baby will be considered full term and weighs around 3 to 4 kg. By this stage the following are fully formed and the baby is ready to take their first breath: brain and nervous system; bones (apart from skull); if it's a boy the testicles begin to descend into the scrotum; digestive system is prepared to cope with breast milk. There is little room for your baby to move, but they will still change position. You may even be able to see them move through your skin!

NB: The skull bones remain soft and separate until after birth so it makes it easier for the baby to travel through the birth canal. They slide over each other, while still protecting the brain.

Weeks 37 to 40

In a few weeks, it will be time to meet your baby, exciting! If it hasn't happened before, then the baby should turn to face downwards and move down into your pelvis, this is called 'engaged'. You may notice your bump move down a little bit. The lanugo should almost have disappeared. The hormones in your system may cause your baby's genitalia to appear swollen when they are born. This will soon settle down. Your baby's digestive system will now contain a substance called 'meconium'. It is sticky and green, and will be your baby's first poo. If your baby does a poo, while you are in labour, the amniotic fluid will have meconium in it. The midwife will want to keep a closer eye on you, as it can mean the baby is in distress.

N.B: If you experience any of the following signs during late pregnancy, make sure you contact your health professional immediately:

- Vaginal bleeding (could signal a serious problem e.g. placental abruption)
- High blood pressure or protein in your urine (pre-eclampsia)
- Itching (at any stage of pregnancy) could indicate a rare pregnancy complication called 'Obstetric Cholestasis'. It is caused by a build-up of bile acids in the blood stream, which causes the itch, and may result in pregnancy complications.

Baby Bath Tub

The Comfort Height Bath Tub offers ultimate comfort for you and your baby during bath time. An extra platform safely raises the tub, making it comfortable and easier to reach baby during bath time.

To Learn More, Go to
www.MillenniumPublishingLtd > Dr-Jane-Smart > Pregnancy Required Items

Chapter 7

Changes During Pregnancy

What happens to your body while pregnant? It is obvious that your body is going through changes but emotions also tend to undergo change, due to the influence of hormones. But how exactly does your body change to accommodate the baby?

Respiratory System

Your respiratory (breathing) system sends oxygenated blood throughout your body to keep vital organs healthy and working correctly. While you are pregnant, you may notice changes to your respiratory system, to compensate for the oxygen demands of your uterus, foetus, and placenta. You may have a feeling of being breathless, from walking or going up-and-down stairs.

Cardiovascular System

During pregnancy, your body needs to adjust to an increased demand on your cardiovascular (heart) system, to meet the demands of both mother and foetus. There is a blood volume increase, of about 40 to 50%, to ensure your baby is receiving sufficient oxygen and nutrients. In addition to the increased blood volume, there is also an increase in maternal heart rate of 15 beats per minute.

Gastrointestinal System

Your uterus increases in size to accommodate an ever-growing baby. It rises from where it usually sits, in the pelvic cavity, and when this happens, your intestines, stomach, and other organs are displaced. The hormone, progesterone causes your lower oesophageal sphincter to relax. This means you may experience: heartburn, constipation and acid reflux.

Endocrine System

Hormonal changes may cause the following:

- Your parathyroid gland increases production of calcium to keep up with you and your baby's demands.
- You may experience hot flushes, thanks to the increase of hormone levels. There is also a significant increase in your basal metabolic rate (the amount of energy the body uses at rest).

- While you are pregnant, the baby's placenta acts as a temporary endocrine gland. This helps produce the large amounts of oestrogen and progesterone your body requires by weeks 10 and 12 of pregnancy. It is also helps to maintain the growth of your uterus and controls uterine activity.

Uterus

Your uterus gradually expands throughout pregnancy. Before pregnancy it is a pear-shaped organ and approximately 4.5cm x 7.6cm and 3cm thick; by 20-22 weeks it reaches the umbilicus (belly button); at full-term it is the size of a watermelon! As you approach your second trimester, you will begin to see changes in your abdomen as your baby grows and your uterus expands to allow the room. It is possible that you may begin to feel an ache, on one side of your abdominal wall, where your ligaments are stretching to support your uterus.

Urinary System

You've probably heard that pregnant women 'wee' what seems like every five minutes! As explained previously, in early pregnancy this is caused by hormonal changes. Later as your uterus expands and exerts pressure on your bladder, pelvic floor muscles, and urethra. You may even experience some leakage of urine when you laugh, cough or sneeze. This is normal and not something to worry about, but be sure to practice your pelvic floor exercises.

Musculoskeletal System

Your bones also change in pregnancy. There is realignment to the curve in your spine, to allow you to keep your balance as your tummy gets bigger. You will feel a shift in posture, that leads to the 'typical gait' you see in women in the late stages of pregnancy. Ligaments become relaxed, due to a hormone called 'relaxin', and this contributes to the back and pubic pain you feel closer to your due date.

Skin

Some women have a certain 'glow' when they get to a point in pregnancy. You may notice hyperpigmentation in a line down the centre of your abdomen (linea nigra), nipples, and even your face. This is caused by hormonal changes that are occurring in your body.

Spider veins

These are small, visible red blood vessels, and do look a little like spiders. They are due to an increase in blood circulating through your body, plus hormonal changes.

Varicose vein

You may get varicose veins during pregnancy, due to an increase in blood volume and your uterus putting pressure on the large vein (inferior vena cava), on the right side of your body. This in turn puts extra pressure on the veins in your legs. Some tips that may help to prevent them are, move regularly, elevate your legs when resting, watch your weight and sleep on your left side.

Stretch marks

These can be common in pregnant women and will most likely occur during the second half of your pregnancy. You will begin to see them on your thighs, abdomen, breasts and even buttocks. Stretch marks are just scars that occur when the skin is stretched beyond what is normal, thanks to the growing baby.

Breasts

Breasts change to allow you to breast feed your baby when they are born (if you so choose). Until your milk comes in after giving birth, you will experience some of these changes, as you progress through pregnancy. Your breasts will become larger and more sensitive, due to the increased levels of oestrogen and progesterone, in your system; your nipples may be more pronounced; the areolas around your nipple will darken and enlarge; colostrum may leak from your nipples; your breasts produce colostrum – this starts in pregnancy and continues in the early days of breastfeeding. Colostrum is low in fat but high in antibodies, protein and calcium and is designed to get your baby off to a healthy start.

Other changes

You may notice an increase in your body temperature in early pregnancy. When you get to around the sixteenth week of gestation, your temperature should start to return to normal.

Cramp in your legs is common, due to fatigue carrying around the extra pregnancy weight. It causes compression in the blood vessels of your legs. This can also occur due to a shortage of calcium, magnesium or an excess of phosphorous.

Thanks to the extra fluid volume in your body, you may also begin to see swelling in your feet and ankles.

Hormones cause changes to your hair/nail texture or growth patterns. You may find your hair and nails grow faster than before you were pregnant.

Nappy Bag

With an artful balance of fashion and function, this modern diaper bag backpack hold all your baby's gear. Perfect for both Mom and Dad, this backpack has all the must-have features of a classic diaper bag including 2 big compartments and 16 pockets for the ultimate organization, easy-grab handles, mommy pocket for your belongings, as well as custom hardware D-rings for stroller (Pram hooks excluded).

To Learn More, Go to

www.MillenniumPublishingLtd > Dr-Jane-Smart > Pregnancy Required Items

Chapter 8

Pregnancy Trimesters

Your baby grows a little every day and your body is designed to keep them safe. During each stage of pregnancy, your body goes through many changes. These changes not only affect you but they have a huge impact on your baby. With each trimester comes new experiences and excitement.

Pregnancy is broken down into three trimesters or stages: First, second and third. Typically, each trimester runs for approximately three months, and the foetal stages and maternal changes will happen accordingly throughout.

First Trimester

The first trimester runs from week 0 through to the end of week 13 (month 0 to 3). Week 1 starts on the first day of your last period and you may not look pregnant but the chances are you may be feeling it. Remember the symptoms from chapter 1, these are when they may occur.

The first trimester is when you officially find out you are pregnant. However, taking care of your body before you conceive is equally important and you should already be taking folic acid. Remember you are not technically pregnant the first two weeks of your pregnancy. The first two weeks consist of your period and ovulation, and your body is preparing itself for the pregnancy process.

It is important to keep a close eye out for any unusual/unexpected symptoms that may occur during this trimester. For example, if you notice significant bleeding, severe dizziness, rapid weight gain/loss, severe abdominal pains please call your midwife/doctor, or visit a nearby hospital immediately!

Second Trimester

This starts at week 14 and runs through to week 27 (month 4 to 6)

This trimester may be the easiest of the three trimesters, as morning sickness will have hopefully have calmed, but is before your baby bump is large enough to cause discomfort.

You may begin to show; you will feel more energetic and the weight gain in this trimester is slow and steady. You may start to experience heartburn and even though you may have cravings you may not be able to indulge them.

If you have not already told family and friends you are pregnant, this may be the time to do so. Your immune system may be a little compromised, so beware of others who are unwell or have infectious illnesses. Due to the increase in the volume of blood in your body, you may experience nosebleeds, gum bleeding, or a stuffy nose.

Third Trimester

The last trimester is week 28 onwards (month 7 to 9). At the end of this trimester you will meet your new baby, however it also comes with its own special set of circumstances.

Your hands, feet, and legs may be swollen due to extra blood volume. But please be aware swelling can sometimes be a sign of preeclampsia, so if you think there is something wrong, contact your health professional immediately.

Your breasts will be larger than normal, this is due to hormonal changes and the production of colostrum. Your breasts may leak, when you least expect it, so it can be handy to have breast pads on hand.

You may experience a 'show' towards the end of pregnancy. This is the mucus plug, that seals the entrance of your uterus, slipping away. It is usually a clear, thick jelly-like substance but can be slightly tinged with blood (or old brown blood). However, if you notice any fresh bleeding with this discharge, contact your midwife/doctor.

Backache caused by your ever-expanding baby bump may be uncomfortable and annoying, and you may feel achy. Sleeping on your side, with a pillow between your knees, can help ease the backache and pains in your body.

Braxton Hicks contractions can be alarming if you don't know what they are. Some women describe Braxton Hicks contractions as a tightening in the abdomen that comes and goes, and that these "false" contractions feel like mild menstrual cramps. Braxton Hicks contractions may be uncomfortable, but they do not cause labour or open the cervix. If you are unsure about your contractions and think they may be real, call you midwife or doctor for advice.

Other symptoms during this trimester include, fatigue, heartburn, constipation, hemorrhoids, shortness of breath, spider and varicose veins, and swelling.

You are probably feeling like you are ready to explode but you are almost there. Your body is preparing for labor and if your baby has yet to turn they may do so now. At week 36, your baby's head has 'engaged' (dropped) and is preparing for its arrival into the world. You could give birth at any moment, so start to prepare things you are going to need for when the baby arrives and decorate the nursery.

Breast Pump

Loved by moms and lactation consultants worldwide, the Spectra S1 Plus Premier RECHARGEABLE Breast Pump is designed to bring confidence and comfort to every moment of the breastfeeding journey. The S1 is portable and quickly rechargeable for active moms, and also quiet and discreet for soothing pumping. The added night light allows you to easily pump at any hour. This pump conveniently weighs only 2.9lbs. With a maximum suction strength of 250mmHg and the ability to be used as a single or double pump, the S1 will be a great asset in your breastfeeding journey.

To Learn More, Go to
www.MillenniumPublishingLtd > Dr-Jane-Smart >
Pregnancy Required Items

Chapter 9

High Risk Pregnancy

High-risk pregnancy is when a condition puts the mother, baby or both at a higher risk. You are more likely to have a high-risk pregnancy if you:

- Are overweight (especially if it is by more than 22kg);
- Smoke;
- Have seizures;
- Have diabetes;
- Use drugs or alcohol;
- Are younger than 18 or older than 35;
- Have a history of genetic defects or
- You are having twins/triplets etc.

Just because you have these factors will not automatically mean you have a high-risk pregnancy and the opposite is true, just because you have no pre-existing health issues will not guarantee a healthy pregnancy. You are also at more risk if you have had any of the above issues/complications in a previous pregnancy.

If you have a pre-existing condition, you need do discuss the pros and cons of pregnancy with your GP and/or supervising consultant. There are many variables to consider and you need an expert to advise you.

Smoking Complications

The nicotine present in cigarettes can stunt your baby's growth, and even a few cigarettes a day means harmful chemicals are reaching your baby. Smoking throughout your pregnancy can cause your baby to have a low birth weight or you may go into premature labour. You are more at risk of suffering a miscarriage, and smoking causes problems with the placenta. Babies are more likely to be ill following delivery; stay longer in hospital or even need care in the special care baby unit.

In addition, smoking during pregnancy and after your baby's birth, puts them at a higher risk of 'Sudden Infant Death Syndrome' (SIDS). Stopping smoking prior to birth is the only safe option for your baby. As soon as you give up, the baby will receive more oxygen.

NB: If you are planning a pregnancy or are pregnant and finding it hard to stop smoking, talk to your doctor about places you can get support

Alcohol

Experts are unsure what is a safe amount of alcohol for pregnant women to drink, so if you are planning a pregnancy, or already pregnant the best advice is to abstain completely. Alcohol is passed from mother to baby, via the placenta, and it can damage and effect the cell growth of the baby (brain cells and spinal cord cells are usually the worst affected). It can cause 'Foetal Alcohol Spectrum Disorders' or the more severe 'Foetal Alcohol Syndrome'. These cause a wide range of behavioral, learning and physical problems, which can vary from mild to severe. If you are having trouble quitting alcohol, talk to your GP, so they can provide the necessary support.

Hyperemesis Gravidarum (HG)

This condition affects about 1% of pregnant women and is an excessive form of nausea and vomiting. It is not known why some women get it and others don't but some evidence shows it runs in families; and if you experienced

HG in a previous pregnancy you are more likely to get it in subsequent ones. Some tips to help alleviate symptoms are:

- Rest;
- Staying hydrated;
- Avoiding nausea triggers;
- Emotional and physical support.

Not all tips work for all women, and it can be a case of trial and error to find the ones that work for you.

Be that as it may, there are medications that can help, including in the early stages of pregnancy e.g. anti-sickness drugs, steroids and vitamins B6 & B12

NB: If you are unable to keep down food and fluids contact your doctor, as you can become dehydrated very quickly when suffering with HG, and you may need to be admitted to hospital for intravenous fluid therapy.

Gestational Diabetes

This is caused because the placenta produces hormones that lead to an increase of sugar in your blood. Your pancreas normally produces enough insulin to control this. If not, then it will cause your blood sugar to rise, and you will develop gestational diabetes. Symptoms may not necessarily arise, but can include: feeling tired; being very thirsty; weeing a lot; a dry mouth; infections like thrush, or blurred vision. Please make an appointment to see your health professional, so you can be monitored more closely. Gestational diabetes may mean you go into premature labour, so your baby will be monitored to make sure they do not show any signs of distress. After birth your baby may need to have blood tests regularly, as they may have low-blood sugar, while they adapt to making the right amount of insulin.

Pre-eclampsia

This affects some women, usually in the second half of their pregnancy, and can even happen after their baby is born. When you see your midwife, they will monitor your blood pressure, and test a urine sample. Pre-eclampsia is one of the things they are checking for. Early signs are high blood pressure and protein found in your urine. Other symptoms include excess swelling of the hands, feet, and legs; severe headaches; vision issues. If you notice any of these symptoms, you need to seek the advice of your midwife or

GP immediately. In most cases pre-eclampsia does not cause any problems, and it improves after delivery.

NB: There is a risk that pre-eclampsia can become 'eclampsia'. These are seizures, that can put both the mother and baby at risk. Contact your GP if you have any concerns.

Ectopic Pregnancy

An ectopic pregnancy can occur when the fertilized egg implants outside of the uterus, usually in the fallopian tube. Symptoms to look out for are:

- A missed period (some women may not know they are pregnant)
- Vaginal bleeding
- Pain in your lower abdomen – on one side;
- Pain in the tip of your shoulder (no one is sure why this occurs);
- Discomfort weeing or peeing.

An ectopic pregnancy may grow large enough that it causes a fallopian tube to rupture. This is an emergency and you need surgery to repair or remove the fallopian tube. Signs of a rupture are: feeling very dizzy or faint; nausea or vomiting; looking very pale; a sharp, sudden, acute pain in your tummy. Seek medical help immediately.

Placenta Previa

This is where the placenta lies unusually low in the uterus, and it may be near or over the surface of the cervix. Early in pregnancy it does not cause a problem, but later it can be an issue, as it will block your baby's way out. They will record the position of your placenta when you have your second scan, and if you are found to have placenta previa they will perform another scan at around the 32-week mark. If the placenta is low it puts you at higher risk of bleeding throughout your pregnancy and labour, and this bleeding may be heavy, which puts you and your baby at risk. Your consultant may recommend that you are admitted to hospital towards the end of your pregnancy, so they can monitor you closely and emergency treatment is at hand. They will recommend you have a caesarian if the placenta is completely blocking your cervix.

NB: If you experience bright red (painless) bleeding during the last few months of pregnancy contact your midwife or doctor immediately.

Placental Abruption

If a placental tear occurs you may notice vaginal bleeding and should seek medical attention. However, approximately 90% of these tears can heal themselves but they may also put you at an increased risk of a miscarriage, premature labour or placental abruption. This is a complication of pregnancy that means the placenta has separated from the wall of the uterus. It can deprive your baby of oxygen and nutrients but also cause severe bleeding that could be dangerous to you both.

NB: if you notice any of the following: vaginal bleeding, abdominal pain, rapid contractions, or your 'baby bump' is tender seek medical attention immediately.

Premature Labour

Premature labour can be divided in groups:

- Extremely premature: under 28 week's gestation
- Very premature: 28 to 32 weeks
- Late prematurity: 32 to 37 weeks

Although it is important a baby gets as close to the due date as possible, sometimes things happen that are outside your control. Some factors mean you may be more at risk of premature labour. These are:

- Multiple pregnancy;

- Lifestyle factors (smoking, recreational drugs, high caffeine intake; poor diet/being underweight);

- Maternal age (under 20, over 35)

- Infections (chlamydia, untreated bladder infection);

- Cervical incompetence (the cervix opens too soon and labour follows).

While some of these cannot be avoided, others can. It is important to receive good antenatal care, have regular checkups and maintain a healthy lifestyle. If you are concerned, contact your GP/midwife immediately.

Social Factors

Older mums

You may hear the term elderly primigravida. This is from the age of 35, so not that old really, but pregnancy from this age may come with additional risks.

Most older mum's these days have chosen to delay pregnancy. Although some women have medical reasons e.g. repeated miscarriages, fertility issues. Many older mum's have chosen to delay pregnancy for social/personal reasons and they tend to be better educated, more confident and financially stable. You do however need to be aware of associated risks, some of which are:

- Decreased fertility;
- Chromosomal abnormalities;
- Developing high blood pressure or diabetes;
- Multiple births;
- Birth intervention (labour induction, forceps);
- Caesarian section.

N.B: It is best to talk to your doctor, before trying to conceive. They can give you a thorough checkup, and advice to ensure you are in good general health, and refer you to a specialist if you have any specific issues that need addressing.

Teen Pregnancy

Most girls usually start their periods about the age of 12, and teen pregnancy is defined as occurring between the age of 13 and 19 years. Teens (both girls and boys) need to be educated to realise that girls can become pregnant as soon as they begin to ovulate, so they need to practice safe sex, if they are to avoid becoming pregnant. If you are a teenager, pregnant and reading this please talk to an adult you trust: mum or dad; school counsellor/teacher, or call a support helpline. Above all you need to get help/advice and medical support for you and your baby, whether you choose to continue with the pregnancy or not.

Bed Rest

For some pregnant woman, they are advised to stay on bed rest (for a short or extended period). They may be at risk of complications such as high blood pressure; pre-eclampsia; vaginal bleeding (placenta previa, placental abruption); premature labour; threatened miscarriage; cervical insufficiency, or there may be growth issues with the baby.

Some women may need to reduce their activity, or reduce their stress levels and being put on bed rest is a way to reduce unnecessary physical activities. However, being put on bed rest is not without its own issues. You may be more likely to experience heartburn, constipation, or you may just feel down as your lifestyle is curtailed. If you do find yourself feeling down, or think you me be becoming depressed, make sure to talk to your GP, as soon as possible. Also, ask friends and family to rally round and create a rota to visit you. Just remember to not overdo things!

Sex During Pregnancy

While this book can be handy to have with you, *it should never replace the advice given by your midwife or doctor.* There are so many issues to think about while pregnant and one common question often arises 'is it safe to have sex while pregnant?' The answer is yes, if you've had a healthy pregnancy. The plug of mucus that seals your cervix, protects your baby from infection and the amniotic sac and strong uterine muscles also protect them. The baby can't tell what is going on, and don't worry your partner's penis can't penetrate beyond your vagina!

With that stated, always practice safe sex, if necessary. Just because you can't get pregnant, you can get genital herpes, STDS, etc.

However, now may not be the time to try new, crazy sex positions and even some of your favorite sex positions may not work well for you during pregnancy. A good sex position that allows you and your partner to feel good is with you on top, so no pressure goes on your bump. The following is a list of other sex positions that are comfortable: Side sex from behind, man on top (pillow under your back to lift you up). Once your baby bump starts to appear, it is important to remember not to apply pressure on it. After giving birth, sex should be put on hold until your doctor gives you the ok, typically after your six-week postnatal check. Sex can still be pleasurable during pregnancy, for both you and your partner, you just need to find out what works best for you both.

Oral sex is also fine, both if you are giving or receiving, but please make sure your partner does not blow air into your vagina. In rare cases, it can cause an air bubble (embolus) in your blood stream, which is a life-threatening condition for you and your baby.

Nappy Disposal Bin

Dispose of your diapers the clean and neat way with the Easy Saver Diaper Pail by Safety 1st. The Safety 1st Odorless Diaper Pail keeps the smell of soiled diapers out of the nursery. It is a convenient one step diaper disposal system and requires no twisting and turning - just drop the diaper in and go.

To Learn More, Go to
www.MillenniumPublishingLtd > Dr-Jane-Smart >
Pregnancy Required Items

Chapter 10

What Do I Need to Take Into Hospital

What goes in a hospital bag and when should I get it ready? Regardless of whether you are having a home, hospital or midwifery-unit birth you need to pack a bag, so everything is in one place and in case of emergencies, at least two weeks before your due date. Your midwife will provide you with a list tailored to your specific hospital/midwifery unit, but here are some things that you might want to include.

- Your birth plan, if you have written one.
- Medication/List of medication for any pre-existing conditions/illnesses you may have.
- Things to help you relax, or pass the time (music, magazines).
- Loose and comfy clothing to wear during labour. Natural fibres are a better choice, than man-made, as they let your body breathe more. You will probably need a few changes throughout labour, so make sure to pack about 3 sets. Some women may prefer to be naked throughout labour, but it is probably wise to

pack them just in case. Don't forget to pack a comfortable outfit to wear home!

- About 24 extra-absorbent sanitary pads (Maternity ones with wings are a good idea).
- Sponge/cloth or a water-spray, to help keep you cool during labour.
- Front-opening, or loose-fitting nighty or tops for breastfeeding; 2 or 3 supportive but comfortable bras (make sure to take nursing bras if you are breastfeeding);
- Breast pads.
- At least 5 or 6 pairs of pants.
- Toiletry Bag;
- Towels.
- Dressing gown and slippers
- Clothing (make sure you include a hat) and nappies for the baby.
- A shawl to wrap the baby in.
- A camera to capture those all-important first moments.

Think about getting to and from the hospital, and make sure you have a contingency plan, in case of unexpected problems with transport. Think about the route you will take, to allow for unforeseen holdups e.g. roadworks. Remember, you can always call an ambulance!

NB: make sure you have rear-facing car seat (and you disable any associated air-bags). Please get expert advice, and ensure you are aware of the new, car seat regulations, that come into effect on 1st March 2017.

If you are having a home birth, you will need to discuss this with your midwife, to ensure you have everything required. But at the very least you will need clean linen and towels available for the midwife to use, sanitary pads and clothing for when your baby arrives. You also need to think about where in the home you want to give birth and if you need to hire specialist equipment e.g. a birthing pool.

Many people have mobile phones, but it can be handy to keep a written list of important contact details: Your hospital and midwife phone numbers; your partner/birth partner's phone number; your hospital reference number, as they will ask for this when you phone to say you are on your way.

Home Equipment Considerations

Babies require a lot of attention and come with a lot of baggage, literally! You may be thinking where do I start, as there are many items to buy before your baby is born. If this is your first baby you may want to buy everything in sight, but just be aware you may find you don't need it all straight away. You will find family and friends will want to help…let them!

Below is a list of items you may need immediately:

- Moses basket and stand
- Sheets and waffle blanket
- Changing table
- Baby monitor
- Baby bouncer
- Pram
- Breast feeding pillow (if required)
- Sterilizer and bottles
- Baby formula (if bottle feeding)
- A baby bath
- Nappy bag
- Scented nappy sacs

Possible purchases are:

- Bottle warmer (a jug of hot water will suffice)
- Breast pump
- Nappy bucket (for terry nappies to be collected by an agency)
- Nappy disposal Bin (these are specialist bins that lock odours away!)
- Dummies (if you think you want your baby to have one)

These things can wait to be purchased later:

- Cot
- High chair
- Safety gate and catches
- Buggy

Newborns need a lot of attention. Make sure you gather a supply of necessary equipment a couple of weeks before your due date.

Some of the obvious items your baby will need are:

- Nappies (terry or disposable);
- Baby wipes;
- Baby powder,
- Nappy rash ointment/cream,

- Baby oil/lotion,
- Baby shampoo.

Less obvious items are:

- Nail scissors (specifically for newborns);
- Baby brush;
- Baby thermometer;
- Laundry powder that is hypoallergenic,
- Thermometer for your bathtub (many parent use the elbow in the water technique, satisfactorily), *but whatever you use, be sure to put the cold water in to the bath first then the hot.* This way you avoid the possible risk of burns to the baby,

During the first weeks after your baby's arrival you may not leave the house often to buy all the necessary items, so make sure you accept help when offered. Babies go through tons of nappies but do not overstock, as they change size frequently. If you chose not to breastfeed or cannot, you will need to buy formula milk.

NB: Do not make up bottles with water straight from the tap. It needs to be freshly boiled and left to cool, for no more than 30 minutes before you make up the milk.

You are going to want to buy clothes for your baby but please remember many people may gift you baby clothes. An item you might want to buy is a swaddle blanket, this keeps your baby warm and comfortable after they are born.

Other items to buy include:

- Baby-grows/onesies;
- Socks;
- No-scratch mittens;
- Leggings,
- T-shirts,
- Cardigans/jumpers;
- Coats;
- Hats;
- Bibs;
- Burp cloths/muslins.

Keep in mind that depending when your baby is born, weather plays a factor when deciding which clothes to buy. Babies grow fast so there is no need to buy too many clothes, before they are born.

It's not just your baby that needs things ready at home for after the birth, you will too. Some items are: Nursing bras;

breast pads; sanitary pads; nipple cream; comfy clothing; a supply of nutritious snacks and foods. Yet again, if people offer to cook for you, take them up on the offer! You will more than likely be able to reciprocate one day.

Baby Thermometer

In times of runny noses and feverish foreheads, you need a thermometer you can trust. Thanks to the clinical calibration technology, the iPROVEN thermometer will give you consistent and accurate measurements time after time.

To Learn More, Go to

www.MillenniumPublishingLtd > Dr-Jane-Smart >
Pregnancy Required Items

Chapter 11

48 Frequently Asked Question (With Answers)

1. How do I know if I am ready to get pregnant?

Thinking about if you are ready or not is a big step. When you are properly prepared, then you will be less stressed about what could or could not happen. Before you get pregnant, it is best that you got to your OB/GYN and get a checkup as well as ask any questions that you may have about childbirth and being pregnant. During this checkup, your doctor will switch you off any medications that you may be on that could harm your fetus when you become pregnant. Moreover, they will also give you the information you need when it comes to folic acid, prenatal vitamins, and everything that you need to have or know about in order to prepare your body for conception.

2. How do I know when is the right time for me to get pregnant?

The best time for you to get pregnant is when you are ovulating. Ovulation happens typically *fourteen days* before your next period is set to start (if you are on a regular schedule. This can be difficult to track if your periods are not regular). Most cycles last twenty-four to thirty days and you will begin to ovulate somewhere between day ten and day sixteen.

3. What are the pros and cons of getting pregnant?

Everyone looks at pregnancy differently, so there are going to be different pros and cons for every woman depending on how they look at being pregnant.

A few cons that are quite common amongst mothers are:

- The decisions that you have to make with regards to getting prenatal screenings, what you are going to do with the results, so on and so forth.

- The lack of alcohol. You are not supposed to drink while you are pregnant. Even though some doctors will tell you that it is okay for you to have a glass or two in moderation, there are others who will tell you to stay away from it completely. It is up to you on whether or not you heed their warning.

- How pregnancy is going to affect your body. Yes, your body is going to change because you are having a child that is growing in your womb thus making not only your abdomen extend as they get bigger, but changing things such as how your breasts appear and things like that.

- Mood swings and lack of sleep. Thanks to the amount of hormones that are flooding your system, you may find that you are more irritable at times than others and that you are having problems sleeping when your baby actually gets here.

Some pros are:

- Bigger breasts. As you go through your pregnancy, your breasts are going to grow large due to the milk that is being produced in preparation for the breast feeding process.

- Being spoiled with love and care. Many women experience that their partners, their friends, and their families tend to spoil them when they find out that they are pregnant because everyone is excited for the baby!

- Your hair and nails are going to grow faster thanks to all those hormones (they are not all bad, they just tend to get a little bit irritating when it comes to certain aspects of your pregnancy).

4. What foods do I avoid during pregnancy?

It is suggested that you need to stay away from:

- Fish that contains a lot of mercury. Having large amounts of mercury in your system can actually end up damaging a developing brain.
- You should also stay away from any unpasteurized soft cheeses such as brie, feta, gorgonzola, etc.
- Raw fish such as sushi.
- Cold ready to eat meals like hot dogs or lunch meat because of the listeria that the meat can contain.
- Unpasteurized milk (which is also a source of listeria).
- Alcohol due to the fact that it can interfere with the development of your fetus and even lead to fetal alcohol syndrome.
- Uncooked or cured eggs and meats such as prosciutto, or runny eggs.

- Caffeine however it is okay when you take it in moderate amounts.

5. What foods should I eat while I am pregnant?

Above all you need to follow a healthy diet and your body needs extra vitamins and minerals. Whatever anybody may tell you, you do not need to 'eat for two'. It is advised that you eat an extra 350 to 500 calories (1470 to 2090 kilo-joules) during the 2nd and 3rd trimesters. If your diet is lacking, it may affect the baby's development.

Poor eating habits and gaining excess weight can put you at a higher risk of gestational diabetes, or birth complications. Things such as leafy greens, vegetables, fruits, whole grain breads and cereals are going to be the best option, while you are pregnant. You also need to consume food that contain protein and calcium, such as low fat yogurts, broccoli, eggs, salmon. When it comes to meat, please refer to the section on what not to eat, but above all make sure the meat is cooked thoroughly!

6. Does it matter if I miss a day of my pregnancy vitamins?

Prenatal vitamins are important in helping to bridge the gap in any of the nutrients that you may be missing in your diet. However, if you happen to miss a day or two of your prenatal vitamins, you are not going to find that anything is going to happen to you or your baby. There are some women who never take prenatal vitamins when they are pregnant.

7. What should I do if I become constipated during pregnancy?

Constipation is something that many pregnant women complain about. This is not too uncommon for women during some point in their pregnancy. With all the progesterone in your system, you are going to realize that your muscles are smoothed out and relaxed, and this also affects the digestive tract.

Due to all the progesterone, your food is going to pass through your digestive system slower. Not only that, but taking iron supplements in high doses is going to cause you to have constipation.

In order to combat constipation, you can:

(a) Drink plenty of water

Your urine should look clear. One glass of juice a day will help as well, most particularly prune juice in order to help regulate your digestive system. There have been reports that drinking some sort of warm liquid after you get up will also help to keep you from being constipated.

(b) Eat foods that are high in fiber

This should be things such as whole grain breads and cereals along with brown rice, beans, and fresh vegetables and fruits. You can also include a tablespoon or two of unprocessed wheat bran with your breakfast along with a glass of water to help you get things moving.

(c) Look at your prenatal vitamins

If they contain a high amount of iron, then ask your healthcare provider about switching to a different prenatal that does not have so much iron in it. The only reason that you need a lot of iron is because you are anemic and are needing to increase your iron intake.

(d) Exercise regularly

Doing light exercises such as swimming, yoga, riding a stationary bike, or even walking can help you to ease the pain of constipation and leave you not only feeling better, but feeling healthier.

(e) After you eat, use the bathroom.

Your body knows when you need to get rid of the waste in it; so listen to it. Do not put off going to the bathroom once you feel the need to. Doing this can cause problems later on.

If all else fails, talk to your doctor about prescribing you something that can help or about adding an over the counter fiber supplement or even stool softener to your daily routine.

The only time that you should begin to worry about your constipation is if there are other symptoms with it such as, abdominal pain, you are passing mucus or blood, or you are having constipation and then diarrhea alternating. At this point in time, you need to get in contact with your doctor or other health care provider as it may be a different issue that is causing this.

While you are going to the bathroom, try not to strain. If you strain you can end up causing hemorrhoids or even cause them to worsen if you already have them. This is caused by the swelling of the veins in your rectal area.

Hemorrhoids are painful and uncomfortable, but will end up going away when you give birth to your baby. If you find that the pain is too severe or you are having bleeding from your rectal, you need to call your health care provider to see if there is a more serious issue going on.

8. What exercises can I do while I am pregnant?

While you are pregnant, you are able to do activities such as swimming, walking, a stationary bike, low impact aerobics, a step machine, and even an elliptical machine. You can also do things such as tennis, racquetball and jogging.

However, you need to be careful and talk to your health care provider if you are unsure if you should be doing the activity.

9. What are my exercise limitations while I am pregnant?

Most exercises you are going to be able to do and you are probably going to slow down and change your routines as your abdomen gets bigger. However, you are going to want to avoid things that are going to give you a higher risk of falling or any kind of abdominal injury.

Along with those, you are going to want to avoid any high altitude sports.

10. Can I have sex while I am pregnant?

Yes!

If your partner is scared of having intercourse with you while you are pregnant. Reassure him that he is not going to hurt you or the baby. If he is still unsure about it, then talk to your doctor about ways that you can help calm his fears so you can get back to doing what you want to do.

11. What is first trimester screening?

This is a test that is done early in your pregnancy in order to offer some information about the chromosomal risks for things such as Down syndrome. Testing is done by either a blood test or by an ultrasound exam.

12. What do I do with my first trimester screening results?

Your results are going to tell you if your baby is at risk for Down syndrome. This test does not mean that your child will have Down syndrome, it only tells you the risk of carrying a baby with this genetic condition.

13. What symptoms are normal while I am pregnant?

There are different symptoms that you will experience while you are pregnant, however, some of the symptoms you may experience are:

- Swelling and bloating,
- Acne,
- Cramping,
- Changes in your sleep pattern,
- Sensitivities

14. Is it normal to have extra discharge while pregnant?

Yes. Not only are your hormones sky-rocketing due to your baby, you also have extra blood flow going to your pelvis. There is a high possibility that you are going to notice an increase in discharge as you go through your pregnancy.

If you find that your discharge has a color, an odor, is painful, or is watery, you need to contact your doctor right away. This could mean that you have an infection of some sort that needs to be treated, or even that your water has broken.

15. What can I expect from my emotions?

You can expect your emotions to be all over the place thanks to the hormones that you have in your system. You may feel like laughing one minute and crying the next. This is perfectly normal.

16. How much is your baby growing each month?

Month one:

This is going to be when your embryo is still starting to develop. There are going to be two layers of cells that are going to help to develop all the organs and vital body parts that your baby is going to need in order to survive.

Month two:

At this point, your little one is the size of a kidney bean and will be moving. There will be webbed fingers, but you can very distinctly see that he or she actually has fingers!

Month three:

During this month your baby is going to be around three inches long and is going to have the same weight as a pea pod. Not only that, but his fingerprints have now developed making him his own unique person!

Month four:

Your baby is now about 5.5 inches long and weighs somewhere around five ounces. It is during this month that he is going to begin to have his skeleton harden from the cartilage that makes up our skeleton to the bones that are going to help him hold his shape and move around.

Month five:

Ten and a half inches in length, your baby now has eyelids and eyebrows. He is also able to stretch out his legs (this is where you will probably begin to feel more kicks).

Month six:

The wrinkles on your baby's skin are starting to smooth out as he begins to put on more weight. With that weight gain, your baby now weighs around a pound and a half.

Month seven:

Your baby can now see what is around him and can open and close his eyes. Your baby is around 14 inches long.

Month eight:

As baby fills out to be rounder and more fully developed, your baby now weights around 4.7 pounds. Not only that, but his lungs are now developed and he is able to breath better.

Month nine:

You're now ready for your baby to come any day now! Baby is around twenty and a half inches long and weighs about seven and a half pounds (could be larger, could be smaller). However, your baby is fully developed and ready to be held by you!

17. Why am I always tired?

During the early and late stages of your pregnancy, you may realize that you are more tired because your hormones are working overtime in order to keep up with all the changes that your body is making for both you and the baby.

It is also possible that you are having trouble sleeping at night because of things like having to go pee all the time, heartburn, or even leg cramps.

18. Will my frequent urination stop while I am pregnant?

Your constant need to urinate will ease up after your baby is born. In the days immediately following the baby's birth, you may realize that you are urinating more often because your body is attempting to get rid of all the fluids that your body retained while you were pregnant.

19. Why am I experiencing headaches while I am pregnant?

You may be experiencing headaches that range from mild to intense due to the rise in hormone production. This is your body's way of trying to accommodate the sudden rises in hormones.

Once your body is used to the hormones, your headache should ease up. If they do not, it is best that you talk to your health care provider.

20. Does being pregnant really cause lower back pain?

Yes, pregnancy really does cause lower back pain. This is usually caused because your center of gravity has shifted to the front of your body due to your ever-growing abdomen.

Changing the way that you sit and sleep can help to ease some of the back pain that you are feeling. If you sleep on your side, you may want to place a pillow between your knees.

You may feel an increase in back pain right before you go into labor.

21. How do I treat morning sickness?

It's an unpleasant side effect but your baby is not at increased risk. Most women find it starts to clear up by week 16 to 20. The following may help to reduce the symptoms, sometimes it is a case of trial and error.

- Get plenty of rest: tiredness can increase nausea.

- Ensure you drink plenty of water, to stay hydrated, but sip fluid. Little and often is better than one large drink, you may find you vomit otherwise. Drinks that are very sharp, sweet or too cold can make nausea or sickness worse.

- If you are feeling sick when you wake up, make sure you take your time getting out of bed. If you can, have something to eat prior to doing so e.g. a dry biscuit, toast.

- Eat smaller meals, more regularly. Foods that are high in carbohydrate can help e.g. pasta, bread, crackers. Pregnant women often find savoury foods are tolerated better than spicy or sweet ones. **NB:** Don't stop eating! If you find the nausea and vomiting prevents you eating, you must consult your healthcare professional.

- Avoid smells or foods that make you feel sick. Some women find they prefer eating cold meals to hot ones, as they don't give off as much aroma. Ask someone else to do the cooking. If this is not an option, try to cook bland foods, like pasta, that don't give off too much of a smell and are easy to prepare.

- Sometimes the more you think about nausea the worse it can be, so try to find something distracting to do. Adjusting the clothing you wear can also help. Trade in your tight jeans for ones with a comfortable elastic waistband

- You may find that ginger products help to counteract nausea, but they are not licensed in the UK. Make sure you buy them from a reputable source, like a pharmacy. You might find that ginger biscuits or ginger ale help.

22. How do I know what trimester I am in?

Your first trimester is going to be months one through three. Otherwise known as week zero to week thirteen. The second trimester is week fourteen to week twenty-seven months four to seven. Month seven to nine is the third trimester. This is week twenty-eight to when you give birth.

23. How much weight should I gain while pregnant?

Normal weight gain for a pregnant woman is twenty-five to thirty-five pounds.

Should you be overweight, your weight gain is supposed to be around fifteen to twenty-five pounds.

If you are underweight then it is safe for you to gain twenty-eight to forty pounds.

If you are having multiple births, you should only gain about thirty-five to forty-five pounds.

24. Is gas and indigestion normal while pregnant?

Yes. With the changes in hormones, the efficiency of the gastrointestinal system is lowered. The first sign is going to probably be nausea and morning sickness. As your pregnancy progresses, it can change into acid reflux and indigestion. This is completely normal.

25. When will my morning sickness end?

For most women morning sickness stops at twelve weeks. However, some women end up having morning sickness till the end of their pregnancy.

Morning sickness is not harmful to your or your fetus. It is only harmful if you begin to experience excessive vomiting and find that you are not able to manage to keep your food down.

26. What are activities I should avoid while I am pregnant?

You do not want to change the cat box. Doing this task can actually end up leading to complications for newborns.

- Paint. The exposure to the toxic chemicals is not good for you or baby.

- Get an X-Ray unless you absolutely have to.

- Use a sauna, hot tub or tanning booth.

- Go on rides such as Great American Scream Machine or Tower of Terror.

27. What can I do to relieve or prevent heartburn?

In order to prevent heartburn, you should try and avoid greasy and spicy foods as well as drinks that contain a lot of caffeine. You can also try and eat smaller meals while avoiding having to bend or lay down right after you have eaten.

28. What can I do to relieve or prevent leg cramps?

Make sure that you exercise regularly and are getting plenty of fluids in your system. It is also important that you do not sit in one position for an extended period of time. Massage your legs in order to keep blood flowing and apply heat when you need to relieve a cramp.

29. What can I do to relieve or prevent hemorrhoids?

Drink plenty of fluids and make sure that you have plenty of fiber in your diet. Exercising regularly and avoiding standing or sitting for long periods of time. You can also try and take sitz baths while applying cold compresses to the effect area.

30. What are some of the complications that I can experience while pregnant?

(a) Before Pregnancy:

As you are trying to get pregnant, you need to make sure you talk to your health care provider about any health issues you currently going through or have experienced in order to make sure they do not cause any complications later in your pregnancy.

If the issue is current, then it may require you to change how you and your doctor are treating that issue due to the medication possibly causing an issue later on.

Also, it is important that you identify any issues that you had in previous pregnancies in order to try and get them addressed and possibly avoid them with this pregnancy.

(b) During Pregnancy:

While pregnant, the complications and even the symptoms of these complications can range anywhere from annoying and slightly uncomfortable all the way to something that can be life-threatening.

Not all the symptoms are going to be physical either. There are some mental issues that the mother can have that can end up effecting not only the mother, but the baby as well.

It is vitally important that you keep track of these symptoms and if anything troubling happens or begins to worry you, talk to your health care provider in an effort to try and prevent any further issues.

(c) Pregnancy Complications:

Urinary Tract Infection (UTI): this is a bacterial infection that occurs in your urinary tract. Signs that you have a UTI are:

- Nausea or back pain
- Fever, tiredness, shakiness
- Pressure in your lower stomach
- Urine that smells bad or looks cloudy or reddish
- An urge to use the bathroom often
- Pain or a burning sensation when you use the bathroom.

Should you believe that you have a UTI, it is important that you talk to your doctor about being tested. If you test positive, then your doctor will be able to give you a treatment of antibiotics so that you can kill the infections to make it better in a day or two.

(d) Anemia:

This is when there is a lower number of red blood cells than what you should have in your body. When you are being treated for the underlying cause of anemia, then you will be able to restore the number of healthy red blood cells. There is a possibility that you will feel tired as well as weak should you have anemia. This can be treated by taking folic acid and even iron supplements.

(e) Mental Health Conditions:

You may even experience depression while you are pregnant. If your depression persists throughout your entire pregnancy, you may want to consider talking to a therapist in order to help you get your depression treated. Depression can actually end up causing you to have trouble taking care of your baby after they are born.

A few other complications that you may come across are, obesity and weight gain, infections, high blood pressure, hyperemesis gravidarum (morning sickness/nausea), or GDM (Gestational Diabetes Mellitus).

31. Is bleeding cause for alarm while I am pregnant?

Yes! Bleeding can actually mean that there are complications occurring in your pregnancy and you need to be seen immediately.

Anything from zero to twenty weeks means that you could be having a miscarriage.

Anything between twenty to thirty-seven weeks means that you could be having preterm labor

And at any time it could mean that there are problems with your placenta such as it having separated from the inner wall of your uterus.

32. How bad will my pregnancy dizziness get?

It is a common symptom to feel dizzy while you are pregnant. During your early pregnancy it means that you could have low blood sugar and need to eat something. You may feel dizzy up until you give birth due to your uterus putting pressure on the arteries in your legs. However, always try and eat something to make sure it is not just low blood sugar.

33. How will I know if I am in labor?

You will know you are in labor when you begin to experience

- Strong contractions that are happening at short intervals,
- Your water has broken,
- You are having cramps in your lower back that are not going away,
- You have a blood mucus discharge.

34. How do I know when I am ready to push?

You will push when you are experiencing a contraction after you have fully dilated. Your nurse or doctor will keep track of how far dilated you are and will tell you when it is safe for you to push and when it is not. You will not push when you are not having a contraction because that will just cause your labor to be harder than necessary.

35. How do I know if the time is right to become pregnant?

Having a baby is a big step. If you are properly prepared, then you will find you will be less stressed whilst trying to conceive and during pregnancy. As they say, 'forewarned is forearmed'. Before you try to conceive, it is best to schedule an appointment with your doctor. They can carry out a general health check and it is a chance for you and your partner to ask questions you may have, about pregnancy and childbirth. If you are on any regular medication or have a chronic illness, this is the time to discuss the issue with your doctor and they can arrange for you to see a consultant. Moreover, your doctor can provide you with information in regards to folic acid, antenatal vitamins, and other steps to prepare your body for conception.

36. What other considerations are there before I have a baby?

Every woman looks at pregnancy differently, therefore there will be very individual considerations/reactions. Some women seem to breeze through pregnancy. Others, can experience quite negative feelings, and this can be quite normal. It is a big step to take and there is a lot to consider. Are you going to undergo antenatal screening? If you do and you receive unwelcome results, how are you going to react/what is your next step?

37. What to do if nausea and vomiting become more severe?

If your nausea and vomiting becomes severe and does not respond to the remedies above, you might find your GP prescribes a short course of anti-sickness (antiemetic) medication. Some antihistamines (for allergies) can also help control sickness. Do not take anything unless it has been prescribed especially for you!

N.B: We discussed Hyperemesis Gravidarum in chapter 9. It needs specialist treatment in hospital, so please contact your doctor if you are concerned

38. What supplements should I take before and during pregnancy?

Folic Acid is a must as soon as you plan on becoming pregnant. You need to take 400 micrograms every day, while you are trying to conceive and up until you are 12 weeks. Why? Folic Acid can help to reduce neural tube defects, such as Spina Bifida. Obviously check with your midwife or doctor first but you need to choose an antenatal vitamin that includes: Folic acid, vitamin D, calcium, vitamin C, thiamine, riboflavin, niacin, and vitamin B12.

39. When will I start to feel the baby move?

Baby movement or 'quickening' is usually felt between weeks 16 to 25. In your first pregnancy, it might not be until closer to the 25 weeks. In a woman's second or subsequent pregnancy they may feel it at 13 weeks. Remember every woman is different but if you are at all concerned talk to your midwife or doctor.

40. What medication can I take while I am pregnant?

With any medication in pregnancy, whether supermarket or pharmacy bought you should discuss taking them with your doctor. There are some herbal/alternative remedies that are safe to take whilst pregnant to relieve things such as nausea. Some are not! So please check with your GP/midwife, before taking them. Also, make sure you adhere to the correct dose. Do not take an increased dose, thinking it will be more effective!

41. Why am I experiencing headaches, while pregnant?

In early pregnancy, there is an increase in hormones and blood flow, and this may mean more frequent headaches. Other causes can be stress, low blood sugar, tiredness and dehydration. Later in pregnancy they tend to be caused due to poor posture. Whatever the cause, before you take any medication to combat them, talk to your GP first.

N.B: Headaches in the 3rd trimester can also be caused by pre-eclampsia (discussed in chapter 7), so make sure you attend regular antenatal checkups, and if you are at all concerned contact your midwife or doctor.

42. Why am I getting lower back pain?

Your body produces a hormone (relaxin) that causes the ligaments in your pelvic area to relax. It may also cause ligaments in your spine to loosen, which can cause pain. Your spine supports the extra weight gained in pregnancy, and your growing uterus puts pressure on nerves and blood vessels in your back and pelvis. Your centre of gravity changes due to weight gain later in pregnancy, so you may start to change the way you stand/move to compensate. Trying the following may help: Regular exercise, to strengthen muscles and to improve your flexibility; improved posture (make sure you don't slouch). Changing the way, you sit and sleep can also help to ease any back pain that you are feeling. If you sleep on your side, you may want to try placing a pillow between your knees.

43. Is heartburn and indigestion common while pregnant?

Digestion is slowed down in pregnancy, due to progesterone making muscles smoother. The valve at the top of the oesophagus can also open or leak, which then lets stomach acid flow upwards. In addition, as your uterus grows, it pushes on your stomach causing more pressure on the valve. To help avoid heartburn, try not to eat greasy or spicy foods, and drinks that contain a lot of caffeine. You can also try and eat smaller meals, while avoiding bending or laying down right after you have eaten.

44. Is it normal to have extra discharge while pregnant?

Yes, but it should be thin, white and normally odourless or mild smelling, and is caused by having extra blood flow going to your pelvis. If you find the discharge changes colour, smells, looks unusual, or you experience pain, itching or soreness, contact your GP. It may mean you have thrush, and this is easily treated.

N.B: Do not use tampons whilst pregnant, as more germs may be introduced into your vagina.

45. How can I relieve leg cramps?

No one is exactly sure what causes leg cramps. But there are a few things you can do if you get them:

- Straighten your leg, then (gently) flex your toes and ankles towards your calf.
- Try standing on a cold surface, as this can sometimes stop a spasm

N.B: If the flexing or cold do not work, make sure you see you GP, immediately. In rare instances the pain could be due to a blood clot. Do not massage, as this could make it worse.

46. Can I prevent stretch marks

Stretch marks are caused, in later pregnancy due to changes in elastic tissue that is just below the skin's surface. Genetics can play a part in whether you get them or not. Although you may not be able to avoid them, you may be able to slow them down. No stretch mark cream is going to prevent them but massaging your skin, with an oil or cream can help you to feel good, and it may even encourage new tissue growth.

47. Is it safe to fly while pregnant?

If you are only having one baby, and your pregnancy has been a healthy one, then you can usually fly up until you're 36 weeks pregnant. Some airlines are reluctant to carry women after 28 weeks, due to the risk they may go into premature labour, so check with the individual airline. If you have a high-risk pregnancy, your doctor may advise you not to fly throughout your pregnancy.

48. Can I eat a vegetarian diet whilst pregnant?

Make sure you plan your meals, and eat a variety of healthy, nutritious vegetarian foods, then you should be able to continue. Make sure you consume all the necessary vitamins, minerals, protein and nutrients that you and your baby need. If in doubt, talk to your midwife or doctor.

Conclusion

Through pregnancy, your baby grows a little every day and your body is designed to change and keep them safe. During each stage, you and your baby go through many changes. With each trimester comes new discoveries and the imminent arrival of your little one can be scary, stressful but more than anything - exciting.

During pregnancy and beyond a woman's life changes forever, and hopefully this book has helped you prepare for these changes. It has covered topics such as symptoms of pregnancy, nutrition and risk factors. If you are experiencing unusual or painful symptoms, be sure to contact your midwife/doctor, immediately. If you are planning a pregnancy, hopefully this book will help you to be well prepared for the journey you may someday embark on. More than anything, enjoy your pregnancy and congratulations for that beautiful baby boy or girl!

www.ingramcontent.com/pod-product-compliance
Lightning Source LLC
Chambersburg PA
CBHW050220270326
41914CB00003BA/500